TANTRA
YOGA

Cover & Graphic Design

Mattias Långström

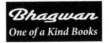

Bhagwan
One of a Kind Books

TANTRA
YOGA

ISBN 9789198735802

✳ ✳ ✳

Publisher: **BHAGWAN 2022**

NAMASTÉ

I want to thank the teachers and students I have had over the years and who have made my journey with yoga so interesting. Thank you for all the inspiration you have given me and for making this book possible. The yoga masters who no longer live among us, live on with every new person who immerses themselves in the yoga tradition.

Sri Swami Sivananda, Sri Swami Satyananda, Sri Tirumalai Krishnamacharya, Sri Swami Vishnudevananda, Sri K. Pattabhi Jois, Osho, Swami Nirdosha, Swami Omananda, Swami Janakananda, Ole Schmidt, Turiya, Maryam Abrishami and Sanna Kuittinen.

Everyone who has searched for answers to what they perceived through an activated ajna chakra. In yoga, they have learned the principles behind the universe, the collective consciousness, and the creative power, Kundalini Shakti. The duality behind everything, both what we see and what we do not see. Together we help to pass on the previous secret knowledge, about our gunas, nadis, and chakras, to anyone who wants to be seen.

THE AUTHOR

Shreyananda Natha is the author of over twelve titles on yoga. Among other things, he has written the most comprehensive books on yoga in Swedish – Everything About Yoga and the study book The Yoga Bible. He is also a certified yoga and meditation teacher according to EYTF's international guidelines and has undergone a multi-year yoga teacher training under the leadership of Swami Omananda at Satyananda Ashram. Shrey-ananda Natha holds the highest initiation in the Tantric Natha Order. He travels frequently to Asia and India to improve himself, and to gain knowledge and inspiration. He has immersed himself in the tantric rituals and is known for his extensive knowledge of yoga, deep relaxa-tion, and meditation

There is no authority that can say what yoga is. When you give yourself fully and completely, and experience yoga without limitations or doubts, when you become one with the true experience in yourself, the real en-counter with yoga arises. Only then do you understand what yoga is – for you. You are no longer limited by ornament, shyness and artificial thought patterns that lie as a filter between you and the transformation. Yoga is a cultural-historical wealth that is still passed on from teacher to student and helps man to find his way back to his true nature. It opens us up and attracts aware-

ness. It strengthens our self-esteem, and our entire person's spectrum of possibilities suddenly becomes visible to us. Yoga is not difficult. You do not have to be vegan or able to stand on your head. You just need to practice your yoga regularly and the rest will come by itself.

With all the love from the universe – Aum Shanti Shreyananda Natha.

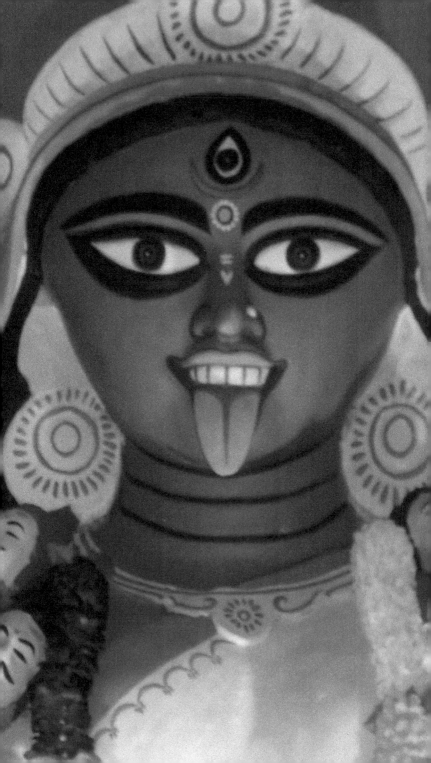

TANTRA YOGA

TANTRA, MANTRA & YANTRA

The word tantra refers to those religious literary works in which mysticism and magic play the main role and form the group of ritual books belonging to the mysticism of later Hinduism.

Tantra books are intended to be a guide in the use of magical and mysterious formulas, and are often in the form of dialogues between Shiva and Durga. The word tantra comes from Sanskrit and is a combination of the words tanoti and trayati, which can be translated as expansion and liberation. Tantra as a method is about expanding the mind and releasing the dormant potential energy that exists in man. Tantra sadhana - different tantric rituals-all evoke Kundalini shakti in different ways.

In order to expand the mind, we must learn not to be controlled by our sensory experiences. When we are controlled by our senses and our ego, we categorize all our experiences into what we "like" and "do not like", which are called raga and dwesha. This categorization leads to suffering and inhibits our development and our ability to see the pure, true knowledge. As we develop and expand the mind, we gradually develop our intuitive ability that is said to be the source of true, eternal, and right knowledge.

In our daily lives, we perceive and take in our surroundings through our senses. If we instead learn to see, feel, listen and turn the mind inwards, we can create an inner experience about ourselves and thus expand the mind. By releasing the energy (Shakti) and merging it with consciousness (Shiva), we create a homogeneous consciousness and experience Kundalini, which is the very purpose of tantra. The difference between tantra and most other spiritual philosophical paths is that in tantra you do not set up a lot of rules that you have to live by.

Everyone has an opportunity to develop, regardless of where they are in their development. One can be sensualist or spiritualist, atheist or theist, poor or rich, strong or weak; the road is for everyone to discover. There are a total of sixty-four different tantras and each one describes a different approach to mind control and expansion. Tantric techniques are often mistaken for being dirty and bizarre when alcohol, drugs and sex are included in certain exercises andrituals. However, it is not used as a means of pleasure but as a means of expanding the mind.

Tantra describes Shakti, the subtle form of energy as a coiled snake at the bottom of the body at the end of the spine, at the Mooladhara chakra. Shiva, the pure consciousness is said to have its seat on top of the head in the Sahasrara chakra. To awaken the Kundalini energy, which in most people is dormant, one must first increase the flow and amount of prana, the vital energy down to the Mooladhara chakra. Then Kundalini shakti can be directed up to Sahasrara chakra. On its way up along the spine, Kundalini shakti passes six chakras or energy pools. When Kundalini shakti rise, they are charged with energy. The chakras act as nodes for our nadis' energy channels, and these vibrate at different intensities. Chakras carry dormant creative forces that are partially evident in our daily lives and whose full potential can only emerge when kundalini shakti have passed through them on their way up to Shiva.

Tantric exercises are divided into three steps in the form of upasana or worship:

Shuddhi – purification of the gross, subtle and psychic elements or tattwas.

Sthiti – enlightenment by concentration achieved by purifying the elements.

Arpana – insight into the cosmic consciousness.

Tantric exercises can be easily distinguished from other non-tantric exercises by the sacred formulas, symbols and rituals used. Through worship and rituals, we want to attract higher subtle forces as well as our inner forces. Tattwa shuddhi belongs to one of the tantric rituals.

FIRST STEP - CLEANING THE ELEMENT

One of the first introductory tantric rituals is tattwa shuddhi, also known as bhuta shuddhi,which aims to purify our elements.

In tantra, tattwa/bhuta shuddhi is used to transform the pranic flow from our elements so it returns to the original unmanifested form – Shakti. As long as the prana flows in our external organs and is fixed in our elements, our consciousness will be limited to the external world. The energy/consciousness is thus fixed and limited to our physical body through our elements. By releasing it, we can also make it expand.

The first step towards expansion is a purification of our basic physical, mental, psychic and pranic structures. In yoga, there are various purifying techniques aimed at this: prana shuddhi, nadi shuddhi, vak shuddhi, manas shuddhi, etc. But the practice of tattwa/bhuta shuddhi, according to the ancient tantras, is comprehensive.

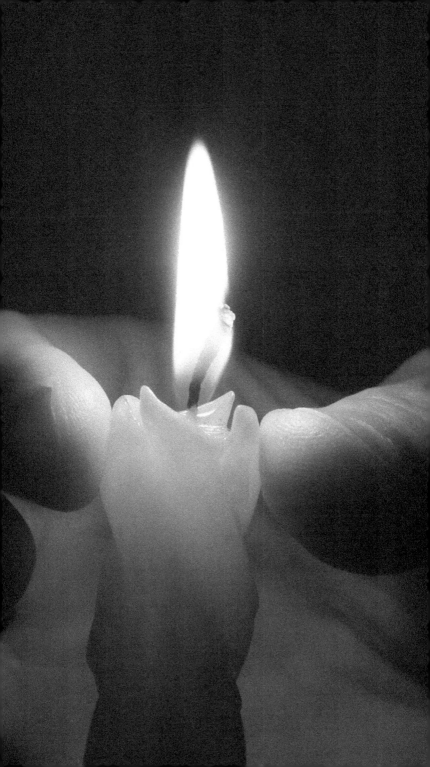

The techniques used in tattwa shuddhi are:

Nyasa – concentration on the body.

Prana prathishta – placement of life and prana in mandala.

Panchopchara – five things sacrificed in the worship of tattwan.

Japa – mantra repetition.

In many of the ancient tantric texts tattwa shuddhi is described as an important technique to move development forward and to gain greater insight. Tattwa shuddhi strengthens our personal experiences of energy and pure consciousness. It is not enough to "know" intellectually that all matter has its origin in the pure consciousness, it must be experienced. The personal experience is the core of tantra and can be made possible with the help of tattwa shuddhi.

By focusing on tattwa yantras, we not only increase the prana in the body but also affect each chakra. Each tattwa is tied to a chakra. Charging each chakra prepares the awakening of the Kundalini shakti and facilitates its path up to the Sahasrara chakra. Tattwa shuddhi *also develops our ability to concentrate (dharana), which leads to spontaneous meditation (dhyana), which in turn leads to awareness of the subtle essence behind matter and form (tattwa jnana).*

BRIEF DESCRIPTION OF TATTWA SHUDDHI

With the help of meditation and self-reflection, the elements that make up the mind and body are purified and transformed. Tattwa shuddhi is a dynamic form of meditation and self-reflection. It is not a passive form where you have to focus on one and the same symbol for a long time. During the implementation of tattwa shuddhi, one easily deepens the mind, by creating images of tattwa yantras (geometric images of the elements), papa purusha (the sinful man) and the mandala of prana shakti (the form of the creative energy).

You start the exercise by creating a mental image of the elements and their respective yantra in the body. You witness how the elements are born from each other and you thus sink deeper into yourself. When one discovers the universal cosmic energy within, one uses the power to heal inner imbalances. With the help of a higher state of consciousness and a stronger and more powerful mind, it is easier to heal imbalances. After this, an inner image of the elements is again created, but in reverse order. Towards the end, one visualizes an image of prana shakti, the energy that is manifested through the elements. Finally, apply bhasma or ash to the body.

Tattwa shuddhi can be used as an aid to entering a meditative state or as a complete sadhana in itself.

To get the most out of the exercise, you should have practiced Hatha yoga and ajapa japa for a long time. The mind and body must be in good condition. You must be able to sit still for a long time without the mind being disturbed by the surroundings. Just before the exercise, it is an important preparation to turn the mind inward which is best done with the help of pranayamas and trataka. You should also have a good knowledge of the location of the chakras in the body and how the prana moves along the sushumna. If you are ill, you should wait until you have recovered before you start practicing tattwa shuddhi.

CLEANING PROCESS

Tattwa shuddhi is a process that cleanses the elements of our body and purifies the senses connected to those elements. The sense of hearing is purified by means of mantra repetition; the sight by observing yantras and mandalas; the feeling and our tactile nerves by applying bhasma or ash to the body; the sense of smell by breathing exercises; and the sense of taste by eating sattvic food or by fasting.

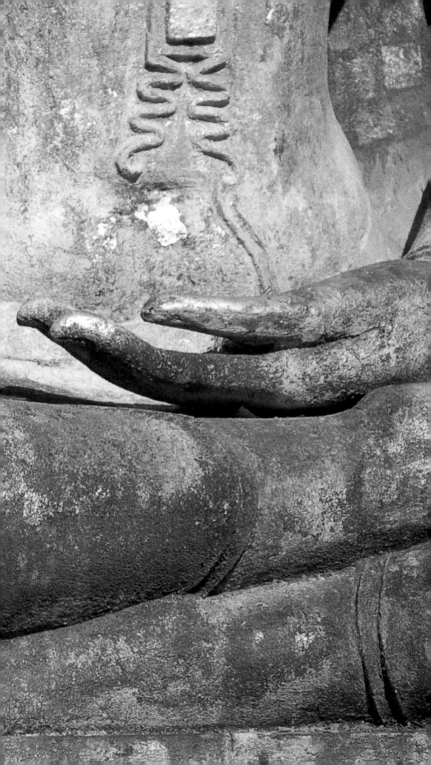

Tattwa shuddhi does not only cleanse our physical body, but cleanses the layers of all of our bodies. In addition to our physical body, we have a number of other bodies relating to the invisible parts of the mind that are affected by samskaras (latent impressions) which create sankalpa and vikalpa (thoughts/counter-thoughts) in our conscious mind.

Imbalances in the various bodies manifest themselves in the form of anxiety, distress, depression, and fear. We often find it difficult to cure these conditions in the same way as physical illnesses. In the long run these imbalances affect our life and our personality. Our body is an extension of our mind and each affects the other. Since the mind largely controls our body and its functions, it is as important to purify your mental mind as it is your physical body.

In tantra, it is said that there is no action or thought that is unclean or wrong in itself. In fact, the unclean lies in wrong perception and judgment. Through sadhanan we can come to an understanding of this and thus fight it. Without purifying the subtle levels of the mind, it is impossible to reach higher levels of consciousness. A mind that is unclean cannot focus or concentrate. By harmonizing the flow of prana in the body, separating the intellect and ego from the consciousness, one can pu-

rify the different levels of the mind so that one becomes the experiencer and the witness at the same time.

CLEANING OF THE ELEMENT

Tattwa shuddhi is a unique technique because it purifies the whole person from the coarsest layers to the most subtle. The first step in the cleansing process is to wash and cleanse the physical body; apply bhasma or ash; and fast and control food intake. Tantra emphasizes the importance of doing all everyday chores with awareness and presence. Everything you do, how you sit, walk, talk, wash yourself, etc. reflects the state of mind. Tattwa shuddhi is thus a purification process that covers all twenty-four hours of the day. However, the first step in the process of physical purity is more about discipline than raising awareness.

The second step in the process purifies the subtle levels. You use your mind and prana. Internal forces are aroused and controlled by the elements. By refining the elements, the energy increases so that they can vibrate harmoniously which creates a balance that leads to an increased inner awareness. By repeating the bija mantra and visualizing the yantra of each tattwa, one can dissolve deeply rooted samskaras and archetypes that prevent us from experiencing the infinite consciousness.

PRANA SHAKTI

In our body, the prana moves in a specific pattern, which means that vibrations are created in different frequency levels. The vibrational frequencies build up our physical body as well as our subtle organs. We can see and feel the physical organs and their constituents while the subtle organs are experienced. In tantra and yoga, these subtle organs are called chakras, nadis, Kundalini shakti, chitta shakti, prana vayu and pancha tattwa.

The prana exists in the microcosm and macrocosm. Without it, we would not function or exist. We would not have the ability to see, hear or move. Most of us have too little flow of prana in our body which leads to fatigue and exhaustion.

The cosmic prana in our body is represented by Kundalini shakti, which has its seat in the Mooladhara chakra. When its full potential is awakened, it rises along the central nervous system of our physical body which in our pranic body is called the sushumna nadi. Kundalini shakti also manifests itself in our larger six chakras.

Each chakra consists of one element. In Mooladhara there are elements of the earth – prithvi tattwa; in Swadhisthana elements of water – apas tattwa; in Manipura elements of fire – agni tattwa; in Anaha-

ta elements of air – vayu tattwa; and in Vishuddhi elements of ether or space – akasha tattwa. The element that controls the chakra reveals the frequency at which the chakra vibrates. Our entire consciousness, thoughts and actions are controlled by the degree of activity of the chakra. Pingala nadi supplies chakras with energy and Kundalini shakti activates and opens them up to their full potential. When our chakras are only partially activated, we become limited in our way of acting and experiencing. In tattwa shuddhi, we affect each chakra directly by concentrating on each tattwa.

MANDALA BY PRANA SHAKTI

In tantra, there is a tradition of symbolizing the various aspects of man in the form of mandalas. Mandalas represent the human subconscious and unconscious mind. By concentrating on these images, we can relax samskaras or archetypes that stand in the way of our creativity and knowledge. In tattwa shuddhi sadhana, an image of prana Shakti is created in the form of a beautiful goddess who has a powerful effect on us.

Prana Shakti as a goddess is red in color. Red is a base color that stands for rajo guna. The color also symbolizes the dynamic quality of prana. Her six arms symbolize the efficiency she has in everything she undertakes. In each hand she holds a tool that all symbolizes different

aspects of human existence. Her three eyes stand for
clairvoyance and the lotus flower on which she sits for
the development of powers and siddhis

ANTAH KARANA

Antah karana is man's inner tool and consists of four
parts: buddhi (intellect), ahamkara (ego), manas
(thoughts and counter-thoughts) and chitta (memory).
According to tantra and yoga, these four are the core of
which consciousness acts from the outside. Antah kara-
na is unique and can only be found in humans. In lower
life forms (animals and plant species) antah karana
exists only in a precursor. Plants and animals act instin-
ctively and not on the basis of ego, intellect or thoughts.
Antah karana is what sets man apart from other species.

Through antah karana, the human consciousness inter-
prets, classifies and perceives everything that concerns
the past, present and future. It can be said that it is a
recipient who receives and sends out impressions. In an-
tah karana, in addition to the knowledge of this life and
what happens here, there is also the knowledge of the
entire universe and cosmos. This knowledge is often un-
manifested and dormant in humans. It is part of human
evolution to refine the frequency of antah karana.

Antah karana is an instrument that we ourselves have

built up through all our incarnations. It carries all the
impressions of our past lives. Antah karana determines
the individual's future actions based on previous expe-
riences and knowledge. These experiences and know-
ledge are often unconscious to us unless we develop our
inner vision and the experience of the cosmos. Through
tantric techniques we can learn to see and control antah
karana which is part of our evolution.

DIMENSIONS OF THE MIND

In yoga, the mind is divided into four parts: jagriti
(conscious mind), swapana (unconscious mind), sush-
pati (subconscious mind) and turya (our transcendental
mind). In modern psychology, only the first three are
mentioned.

Antah karana acts on the basis of the conscious, sub-
conscious and unconscious mind. Manas and chitta,
which are part of the conscious and subconscious mind,
control thoughts and actions on the conscious and sub-
conscious plane. Buddhi and ahamkara constantly exist
to varying degrees in the conscious, subconscious and
unconscious mind. Since all of these have arisen from
the same principle, which is Shakti, they influence each
other intensively.

The three gunas, sattva, rajas and tamas lay the foun-

dation for antah karana. These three cosmic principles have a great influence on manas, chitta and buddhi and thus affect our experiences. The fourth sense, turya is not affected by the interplay between the three gunas. Turya can only be developed by refining antah karana through sadhana. In tattwa shuddhi we learn to perceive antah karana and use its full potential for further spiritual development.

BUDDHI

Buddhi is the principle that most closely resembles pure consciousness. It motivates us to follow our dharma. A sattvic buddhi is characterized by wisdom, happiness, perseverance, calm, self-control and discernment. Under the influence of rajas, some defects occur, which means that the ability to distinguish deteriorates and even actions are affected by wrong knowledge and avidya. A tamasic buddhi acts under the ego, is judgmental and permeated by misinterpretations of the outside world. In tattwa shuddhi, the principle of buddhi is meditated on sattvic. This removes the qualities of rajas and tamas that stand in the way of a sattvic buddhi.

AHAMKARA

Aham means "I" and ahamkara is the ego or what one experiences as the "self". The ego is the core of individualism, which makes us identify with matter. Ahamkara *is very subtle which makes man get stuck in its net life after life. At the same time as the ego binds man to objective experiences, it is the core that must be opened in order to experience unity. Without the ego, man would not be aware of his existence. On the conscious plane, the ego acts through our physical body, senses and mind. On the subconscious plane, it acts through our astral body and dreams. During deep sleep, the ego withdraws while during meditation it functions as the inner consciousness.*

A sattvic ahamkara acts as a catalyst for self-realization. Ahamkara usually takes up the comrades' and underlying experiences from the subconscious mind, but in a sattvic state this stops. A rajasic ahamkara raises the identification with the "self" and leads to restlessness and a constant need to do something. A tamasic ahamkara strengthens painful and negative samskaras which causes fear and doubt. Through tattwa shuddhi we can learn to see how the ego works and thus stop identifying with it.

MANAS AND CHITTA
Manas and chitta represent the external mind: thoughts that come up in our waking state as well as during dreams. Chitta is the core of all experiences in the form of samskaras, archetypes and memories. Manas, i.e. our

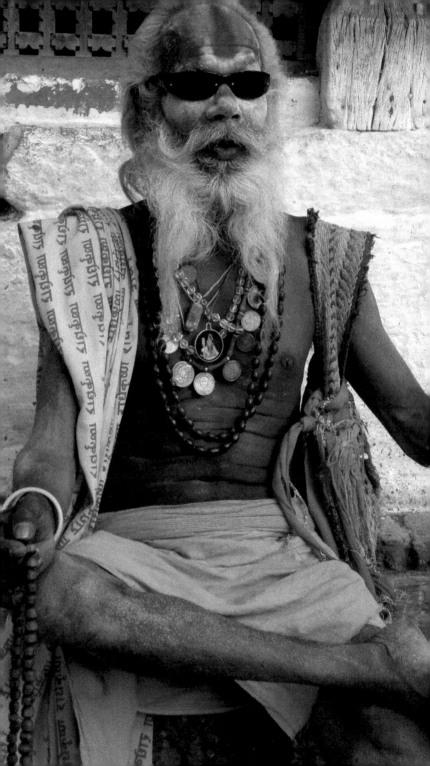

thoughts, are chitta's tools that coexist, and by which archetypes and memories are expressed. Manas and chitta do not work individually but are influenced by both buddhi and ahamkara. In a sattvic state, our manas are steady, focused and concentrated. Under the influence of rajas our senses are activated which creates an imbalance in our intellect. A tamasic manas makes the intellect and the senses sluggish and inactive.

When chitta is in a sattvic state, our senses are withdrawn so that consciousness remains undisturbed. Under the influence of rajas, rajasic is awakened samskaras in chitta in the form of vikalpa (fantasy) and viparayaya (wrong knowledge). In that state, chitta contains both types of cohabitation, knowledge and ignorance, passion and freedom. When tamas prevail in chitta, unwanted samskaras will come up in the form of vasanas (deep-rooted desires).

Coexistence of a negative nature can only be eliminated through reflection, dharana and dhyana. Tattwa shuddhi helps us to enter into meditation which has the purpose of liberating the consciousness. Only then can we reflect on the structure of the elements and influence them.

PANCHA TATTWA – THE FIVE ELEMENTS

All matter is made up of the five elements, akasha, vayu, agni, apas and prithvi. The elements lay the foundation for creation and make it last. The elements affect every aspect of our life, thoughts and actions. In yoga, it is important to learn how these elements work in order to be able to control and influence them and our lives. In tantric texts, the science behind the elements is described.

The elements form a kind of chain where they are born from each other. Akasha is the first element of the process. Akasha consists of subtle matter and energy, which rests in consciousness. When the energy in akasha begins to vibrate, movement is created, vayu tattwa starts to take shape. Vayu stands for the movement that permeates everything. The intense movement creates heat, which causes the next element in the joint (agni) to be created. Agni tattwa has a slower vibration than vayu. This allows the heat to cool down and form apas, the elements of water. The vibration and movement of the apas is minimal. The last element, prithvi, occurs when the movement/vibration is further reduced. Apas solidify and become the elements of the earth. The elements should be seen as an extension of pure consciousness, not as separate existing parts.

During evolution, tattwas have been further developed through tanmatras. Tanmatra is the quality through which tattwas are perceived. Akasha is perceived through shaba tanmatra (sound), vayu through sparsha tanmatra (feeling), agni through roopa tanmatra (vision), apas through rasa tanmatra (taste) and prithvi through gandha tanmatra (smell). When we are born, we are created from the roughest form of the elements. In tattwa shuddhi we create an experience of the elements in their subtle form in order to develop spiritually.

The Patanjali Yoga Sutras state that each element consists of five different characters. To take control of the elements one must practice samyama which is a combination of concentration, meditation and samadhi. Patanjali called this bhuta jaya, "knowledge of the elements". The first character of the five elements is the rough form that relates to experiences that we take in through our senses: sound, touch, form, taste and smell. The second character relates to the quality of the elements: the liquid property of water, the heat of fire, the movement of air and the space of ether. The third character is the subtle form of tanmatras. Here, tattwas are experienced in the form of subtle sounds, sensations, form, smell and taste and are often called mental visions. The fourth aspect of the elements relates to the three gunas(sattva, rajas and tamas) which are an essential part of the elements. One should strive to transform the qualities of rajasic and tamasic into more sattvic in order to develop spiritually. Tattwa shuddhi enables this change. The fifth aspect of the elements is called arthavattwa which stands for the actual goal of the elements. The scriptures describe that it is for the liberation and enjoyment of consciousness from matter that the elements have developed.

The elements are characterized by shaba (sound) and warn (color) and are created by the vibration in the element. The color refers to the energy frequency of the element. Akasha is black in color as the vibration is minimal. Vayu vibrates in the frequency of blue, agni in red, apas in white and prithvi in yellow. The second manifestation of energy of the elements is sound in the form of bija mantras. Bija mantra for akasha is Ham, for vayu – Yam, agni – Ram, apas – Vam and for prithvi – Lam.

Sound and color together builds the form of energy. Akasha is experienced as a circle, vayu as a hexagon, agni as an inverted triangle, apas as a horizontal crescent moon and prithvi as a yellow square.

AKASHA TATTWA – the element of space.
Akasha can be described as the space or emptiness

between two objects or matter. Akasha is the most subtle of all the elements and is almost motionless. It stands for the whole spectrum of sounds, from the rough to the subtle and acts as a carrier for the sound. The vibration of the element is so subtle that it cannot be experienced with external senses. It is said that ether moves at a higher speed than sound. Akasha tattwa is boundless and permeates the entire cosmos, therefore it has the shape of a circle. It is not of matter as we know it and cannot be experienced physically. Tattwa jnanis has discovered akasha by refining the rough mind. Because of this quality, tantra has described the element as mental in nature (not physical) and as the "space of the mind" behind closed eyes, which is called chidakasha. Tattwa akasha stands for the space in the body between our organs. On a mental level, tattwa akasha controls the emotions and passions of man. The best time for meditation and concentration is when akasha flows in the body, which happens about five minutes every hour. The element has its seat on top of the head. Mentally it relates to our unconscious mind and its psychic centers are the Vishuddhi chakra. The spiritual experience created by the element is jnana loka and anandamaya kosha.

VAYU TATTWA *– the element of air.*
Vayu can be translated as air. The element is gray-blue and is symbolized by a hexagon. Vayu stands for

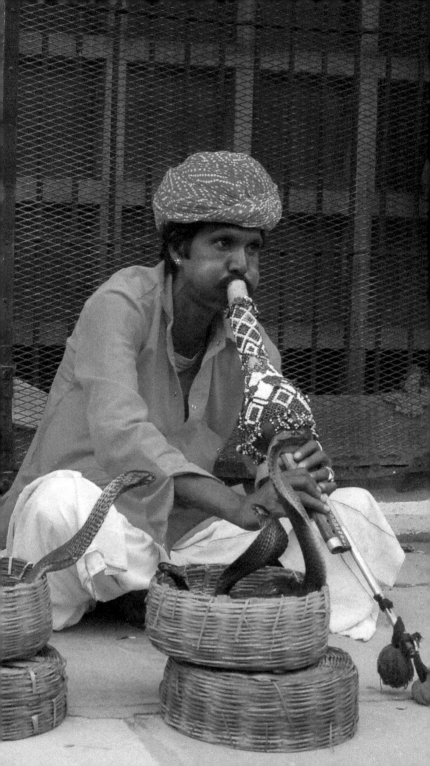

*kinetic energy in all its forms: electrical, chemical, vital
and prana. Its quality is movement and it controls all
movement qualities in the body which consist of prana,
apana, samana, udana and vyana. Vayu is responsible
for our ability to experience physical touch. When we
develop the mind for touch, we can experience the
feeling of energy in us and around us. Even vayu is
physically invisible. The element can be described as
"energy in motion". Movement creates change, which
means that this element can cause stability and instability both in humans and in the environment. Vayu has
its seat between the heart and the eyebrows. Mentally,
the element relates to the subconscious mind. Its psychic
centers are the Anahata chakra. The spiritual experience of vayu is maha loka and vijnamaya kosha, our
intuitive body.*

AGNI TATTWA – *the element of fire.*
*Agni or fire is known as tejas which means "to sharpen".
The element is primarily energy and is experienced as
light. With the help of light we can see the shape. The
sense organ that agni relates to is the eye and it gives us
the ability to see. Form or matter is the core of the emer-
gence of our ego. The ego identifies with form, which
leads to attachment to things. Agni tattwa is thus not
only the first manifestation of the form but also the stage
when ahamkara begins to grow. The element wears the*

color red, which indicates fire and heat. The yantra is a red triangle. Agni is often called the "devouring force" and stands for instability. The power of fire is destructive but can be seen as a catalyst for change, development and evolution. In our physical body, tattwa agni regulates our digestive fire, appetite, thirst and sleep. It has its place between the heart and the navel. Its psychic centers are the Manipura chakra. The spiritual experience of the element is swar loka and manomaya kosha, our mental / thought body.

APAS TATTWA – *the element of water.*
Apas can be described as a large amount of intensively active matter that has emerged from agni tattwa. It is matter that is not yet coherent as the molecules and atoms are in great chaos. It is said that the universe takes the form of tattwa apas before it appears. Yantra for the element is a horizontal crescent surrounded by water. In our physical body we can see apas in the form of blood, mucus, bile and lymph fluid as it controls our body fluids. The element affects our thoughts related to ourselves and worldly things. The apas has its seat between the navel and the knees. Mentally, it relates to our subconscious and conscious mind. Its psychic centers are the Swadhisthana chakra. The spiritual experience of tattwat is bhuvar loka and pranamaya kosha, our energy body.

PRITHVI TATTWA – *the element of earth.*

The last tattwat is prithvi which is also called bhumi, "to be". In prithvi, the motion of the particles has stopped almost completely. Energy has become matter in solid, liquid or gas form. This element bears the yellow color and the yantra is a yellow square. It has the qualities of firmness, weight and cohesion. In our physical body we can see this in the form of bones and other organs. Since prithvi has emerged from all the other elements, it has all the qualities in itself, but the smell is the dominant quality. The element creates stability physically, mentally and in our environment and stands for the material. It has its physical place between our toes and knees. Mentally, it relates to the conscious and subconscious mind. Its psychic centers are the Mooladhara chakra. The spiritual experience of tattwa is bhu loka and annamaya kosha, our physical body.

TATTWAS AND KOSHAS

The elements build up layers that in yoga are called koshas. Man is said to be made up of five different layers, all of which vibrate differently and relate to different levels of consciousness. The first and coarsest layer is called annamaya kosha which is our physical body and which is made up of food. Pranamaya kosha is the layer of prana, manomaya kosha is the layer of thoughts, vijnamaya kosha is the layer of intuition and the last layer is the layer of body bliss, anandamaya kosha.

These subtle layers of man can only be affected with the help of yoga, tantra and other spiritual exercises. In tattwa shuddhi, annamaya kosha and pranamaya kosha are affected by controlling respiration and increasing the flow of prana. Manomaya kosha is affected by concentration. Vijnamaya kosha is aroused by concentration on tattwa yantras. There is no direct exercise to influence anandamaya kosha. It is necessary to work with the other four layers of bodies to get an experience of anandamaya kosha.

Experiences of color, light and smell that come up during tattwa shuddhi are experiences of our subtle bodies.

Koshas are also linked to seven planes of consciousness. These are called lokas. Each loka relates to a plane of existence through which consciousness develops. The elements have an influence on each loka and through tattwa shuddhi we also influence these.

TATTWAS AND BREATHING
In our physical body, elements such as chitta shakti, prana shakti and atma shakti are manifested. These act in the body and mind through our energy channels, nadis or breathing (swara). Swara and nadi mean flow. Nadi is the flow of shakti in our subtle body while swara shastra is the flow of our breathing in nadis. Swara shastra is

thus the science behind the flow of breathing and nadis. The three shakti that flow in our breath are channeled through three main nadis in the body (ida, pingala and sushumna). It is said that we have about seventy-two thousand nadis in the body. Ida, pingala and sushumna are responsible for the psychosomatic and spiritual part of the body, mind and consciousness.

Chitta shakti, which is the power of ida nadi, is our vital and mental energy that controls all our functions regarding thoughts, mind and chitta. All mental activity is the result of the flow of ida. This flow is connected to our left nostril and affects our right side of the brain. It is also called chandra swara and relates to the negative aspect of the energy in the body.

Prana shakti flows through the pingala nadi. It is the vital life energy and relates to the positive aspect of it. All physical activity is controlled by prana shakti. The flow of pingala nadi is connected to our right nostril and affects the left side of the cerebral hemisphere. It is also called surya swara. Atma shakti is channeled through sushumna nadi. Pranan's central passage for spiritual consciousness. Sushumna is neutral energy and is active when breathing flows through both nostrils at the same time. This condition affects the activity of the dormant parts of the brain. In our physical body, these three nadis relate to the parasympathetic (ida), sympathetic (pingala) and autonomic (sushumna) nervous systems. In most people, sushumna is closed for most of their lives, which means that they are controlled by ida and pingala. Through yogic and tantric exercises, one can open up sushumna nadi.

These three aspects of energy manifest in our breathing cycles. The flow lasts about an hour in each nostril. When the flow changes, the sushumna is open for a few seconds. In our flow of swara, the elements are included. Each element has a specific pranic frequency and affects various bodily functions. Tattwas cause the swara to flow in different directions and affect ida, pingala and sushumna. Ida and pingala nadi channel shakti to the chakras in the body and affect their vibration. The elements also affect the chakras in the body through breathing. Each chakra is dominated by one element – Mooladhara by the earth element, Swadhisthana by the water element, Manipura by the fire element, Anahata by the air element and Vishuddhi by the air element. Just as breathing affects our mental, physical and spiritual existence, so do the elements through their different character affect our state of mind, body and consciousness.

Through various tantric and yogic techniques, it is

*possible to practice the feeling for which tattwa is active
in the swara for the moment. A tattwa yogi can in this
way assess his physical, mental, emotional and spiritual
condition. Examples of exercises that practice the ability
are trataka on tattwa yantras as well as sensations of
the elements (color and shape) during the performance
of naumukhi mudra, yoni mudra or shanmukhi mudra.
The last mentioned exercises practice our knowledge
and experience of the elements as they work. You close
the gates for external perception and at the same time
open up to the inner experience of color, sound, smell
and form.*

MANTRA, YANTRA & MANDALA

*The theory and philosophy behind tantra are closely
intertwined with mantra, yantra and mandala. Tantra
is both a philosophical and practical science where
its sublime theories become effective through the use
of mantra, yantra and mandala. The unique thing
about tantra is that there is always an explanation and
practical exercise for each philosophy or theory. Mantra,
yantra and mandala are used in all tantric exercises.
Also within tattwa shuddhi.*

MANDALA

*The word mandala means circle, and in Hindu and
Buddhist rituals it refers to a figure drawn on the*

ground or painted on a table and symbolizes the cosmic and celestial regions. Mandala is a kind of meditation figure constructed of circles and shapes. Properly depicted and properly inaugurated, it becomes a concentrate of occult energy, which attracts hidden forces and itself emits rays like a talisman. Within the boundaries of the mandala circle, other geometric figures are drawn: smaller squares, triangles and circles that divide it all into sacred zones.

To be able to create a mandala, one must be able to see into oneself. Not by thinking – but by vision, as clearly and distinctly as with open eyes. The clearer the inner vision, the more powerful the mandala that is created. The principle behind a mandala is that it exists in the form of a circle. The circle stands for the basic shape behind everything. Anything can shape a mandala, a tree, a house, a car, an animal, a human being. Even the body is a mandala. To be able to create a mandala that carries strength and power, one must have the ability to create an exact copy of the inner vision. Mandala is the essence of an object experienced by someone who has refined the inner vision, an inner cosmic image of which everyone can partake. The level of consciousness lays the foundation for what the mandala will look like. All forms of art, sculpture and architecture are from the beginning mandala's given form.

In tantra, mandalas are also depicted in the form of illustrated images of divine forces. A human form of the divine makes it easier for the rough mind of man to understand and experience the power within, when the ability to visualize is weak. The symbolism and structure behind the images of deities are intended to awaken the equivalent in the consciousness of the individual. By concentrating on mandalas, deeply rooted samskaras are awakened within.

Perhaps the most talked about mandala created in tantra is maithuna kriya. Maithuna kriya forms a mandala that has corresponding yantras and mantras. The erotic sculptures of the Khajuraho Temple in Orissa are based on the tantric belief that maithuna is an act intended to awaken the divine forces in man. The man represents Shiva, the physical energy, and the woman represents Shakti, the mental energy. Through their exoteric and esoteric union, mandalas are created in the form of a force field or energy circle. Linga and yoni mandala are also symbols of this higher union. Man and woman physically unite with each other to re-experience the unity from which they were created. This union is an inner experience in the same way as the spiritual experience.

YANTRA
A yantra is an abstract mathematical image of an

inner vision. Behind each rough shape is a subtle shape, which the yantra represents. Everything in nature can be experienced in its original form (yantra). It carries an inherent energy just like everything else in creation. By visualizing and concentrating on the yantra, one can awaken the corresponding energy in oneself. The yantra is made up of the basic and original shapes: bindu/dot, a circle, a square and a triangle. Bindu is the point from which everything has been created and to which everything will return; it is the process of creation and dissolution. It also represents the union between Shiva and Shakti. Bindu is also found in our physical body, on the top of the back of the head and is called bindu visarga. During meditation, one uses the outer bindu in the form of a yantra, in order to experience the contraction of time and space in bindu in the physical body. The triangle stands for the first shape that comes out of creation and is also known as the moola tricona (spelling should be trikona in English). Upside down it stands for Prakriti (creation) and with the tip facing upwards it stands for Purusha (consciousness). The circle represents the cycle of timelessness where neither the beginning nor the end exist, only eternity. This symbolizes the process of birth, life and death. The square is the base on which the yantra rests and represents the physical, earthly world that must be refined.

Yantras create a path from the outer to our inner. They are of great importance for our continued spiritual evolution: they strengthen our creative and intuitive sides, as well as our spiritual experiences. In tattwa shuddhi, one uses yantra created from the four basic forms.

MANTRA

In the same way that every thought has an equivalent in the form of an image, every image also has an equivalent in the form of sound, nada or vibration. These sounds are called mantras. Mantra means "contemplating what leads to liberation". Nada is one of the first manifestations of creation, the form. In Indian philosophy it is believed that the first sound of creation was the sound of "Om" which is the cosmic mantra. Mandukyo upanishad describes how the mantra effects and expands different levels of consciousness. "Om" is made up of three syllables "A", "U" and "M" which all vibrate at different frequencies which affect the consciousness in different ways. When you repeat "Om", you raise awareness to the same frequency as the mantra. This applies to all mantras.

Nada consists of four frequencies: para (cosmic), pashyanti (temporary), madhyama (subtle) and vaikhari (rough) and correspond to the four frequency levels that "Om" carries: consciously, unconsciously, subconscio-

usly and turya. The entire Sanskrit alphabet consists of mantras. In Sanskrit, the letters are not called letters but akshara, which means imperishable. Each akshara can be used as a mantra. Therefore, it is said that only by reading vedas can one achieve liberation.

The most powerful form of mantra is the bija mantra. Bija means seed and is the sound from which all other mantras are derived. Bija mantra is a powerful, concentrated energy attributed to different levels of consciousness. In tattwa shuddhi, bija mantras are used that relate to the five elements. Even in tantra, it is known that each physical body part has a mantra to which it corresponds. These mantras are used in nyasa to transform the physical body into a container for greater powers, which is aroused by tattwa shuddhi and other esoteric techniques.

Breathing has its own mantra created by the sound of inhaling (So Ham) and exhaling (Ham So) and is known as the ajapa japa mantra. In the upanishads it is said that this mantra is powerful enough in itself to be able to awaken Kundalini shakti and expand consciousness. In the introduction to tattwa shuddhi, the mantra So Ham is used to create a sense of belonging to the universal consciousness.

By repeating the mantra you raise the consciousness, and by concentrating on a yantra you focus the consciousness to a point. At a level of consciousness the inner experience manifests itself in the form of a thought or emotion, at a higher level it becomes an inner vision or mandala. When you go deeper, it turns into a yantra that is later manifested as sound, nada or mantra. When the mind functions under lower and coarser frequencies of energy, it becomes static, sluggish, slow and tamasic. When you make the energy more subtle through mantra, yantra and mandala, the state of mind changes from tamasic to becoming rajasic and finally sattvic.

Mantras, yantras and mandalas used in tattwa shuddhi have nothing to do with religion, occultism or mysticism. They should be regarded as highly charged forces whose intention is to create the same frequency in man that the mantra, yantra or mandala itself carries in order to raise consciousness.

VISUALIZATION AND FANTASY
To be able to create, one must first and foremost have the ability to visualize and fantasize. The imagination is a mental ability that can be used in all ways. When you create an inner world of visions and symbols, the power of the mind becomes stronger. In tantra, visualization

*and imagination create a link between the objective
and subjective worlds. Tantric visualizations serve as a
guide for the practitioner, a medium to concentrate on.
In tattwa shuddhi you want to make the practitioner
experience their inner self through the creation of colors,
sounds and images, and visualization of these in concre-
te form. The pictures are both grotesque and pleasant in
nature. The practitioner has clear guidelines to follow to
help him reach deeper. In the beginning, you experience
the images in the form of thoughts, which over time
develop into clear, inner images.*

THE PERFORMANCE OF PAPA PURUSHA
– the sinful man.

*The meditation exercises in tattwa shuddhi consist of
many unusual fantasies. The most bizarre of these is
papa purusha. Papa purusha symbolizes the cause of
suffering, conflict, disharmony and imbalance caused
by ego, jealousy, pride, etc. During the exercise, you
imagine how papa purusha is transformed and takes
shape, which means that you transform yourself. Papa
purusha's transformation refers to the inner transformation. The transformation and conflict between the
negative and positive forces (ida and pingala) which
constantly strive to unite and transform into the third
neutral force. This conflict acts as a catalyst for our evo-*

*lution and causes us to continue to seek balance in life.
In our search for balance, we turn to the spiritual paths,
which guide our evolution further and further forward.
Without the conflict between the opposites of energies,
we would remain complacent and lazy. Tantra emphasizes the importance of experiencing conflict in order to
create harmony.*

*The performance of papa purusha is covered in the stage
during the exercise when you have become the experience. You witness every action and thought. Each reaction
is assessed objectively. It is only then, when one can look
at oneself objectively, that one can see the sides of one's
personality that the ego has previously hidden; ages you
would rather not see or know about. Here, too, Tantra
emphasizes the importance of daring to see oneself as
one is, not as one wants to be. Only then do you have
the opportunity to change yourself.*

BHASMA

*Tattwa shuddhi includes a symbolic act where one lubri-
cates the body with ash (bhasma) to cleanse the body
physically as well as subtly. The great yogi Shiva, who
is the father of tantra, is often depicted sitting naked
anointed in ashes. Lubricating oneself with bhasma is
considered to favor the experience and discovery of one's
own Shiva nature.*

Bhasma means "dissolution" or "decomposition" and refers to a decomposition of matter by means of fire or water. The "bhasmatic" form of matter is produced, which is considered to be a purer and finer form than the original and all impurities disappear. All matter must undergo this process in order to finally be transformed into the fine essential form. This also applies to us humans. To cleanse means the elimination of slag and impurities. The application of bhasma symbolizes the journey that our inner consciousness makes from the rough matter to the pure consciousness.

Bhasma is also used in Ayurveda as a medical treatment method. Bhasma can be made of gold, silver, copper or other metals. In tattwa shuddhi, cow dung is used. The use of cow dung in India is common as they are considered antibacterial and antiviral as well as generally beneficial to the skin. The reason why you use cow dung in tattwa shuddhi and no other substance is important. By dissolving the cow dung with the help of agni (fire) one reduces it to its bhasmatic form which symbolizes the dissolution of our senses which we try to do in tattwa shuddhi. Through pratyahara we loosen up the experience of the objective world, our surroundings. Through dharana we concentrate the experience of what is left to experience and through dhyana we broaden this experience to its original cosmic essence, the Shiva-consciousness.

*In tattwa shuddhi, bhasma is applied to the forehead
at the same time as the mantra is pronounced, towards
the end of the exercise. Most people who have done this
experience a feeling of having been deeply cleansed.
Rishis and yogis have used bhasma throughout the ages
and its beneficial effect has led to the technology being
used even today.*

THE EFFECT OF TATTWA SHUDDHI SADHANA

*The effects of tattwa shuddhi are faster and more power-
ful when compared to other sadhana, as it is a tantric
upasana that one dedicates to Shakti, the energy principle behind everything. The effects manifest themselves
both materially and as mental forces (siddhis). However,
it is important to keep in mind to perform tattwa
shuddhi correctly so as not to create imbalances and
obstacles that interfere with the continued spiritual development. It is important to learn the technique from a
knowledgeable teacher or guru. Regularity is important
for the exercise, not how often you practice. In tantra we
want to train the mind, intellect and consciousness. We
want to be able to control it with our own willpower. To
teach us that, regular practice is important.*

PHYSICALLY

*The combination of fasting and tattwa shuddhi contri-
butes to changes throughout our physical body. When*

we cleanse the elements (tattwas) that our body is built of, our heart, liver, kidneys, pancreas and all other organs are affected. Tissues and cells are renewed and given new energy, which contributes to a healthier body and mind. Bhasma has a cooling effect on the body and nervous system, which can be heated during intense meditation.

MENTALLY

By visualizing and concentrating on tattwa yantras, chanta mantras and creating mandalas, we purify samskaras that can be manifested through dreams, visions and thoughts in our conscious mind. Mental visions are a common effect of most yogic exercises, but within tattwa shuddhi these are usually stronger when one has developed a sharp inner consciousness. You can experience these as subtle sounds, smells, as a feeling on the skin, or as taste and shape.

SIDDHIS

Yoga shastras clearly describe that siddhis can be achieved by concentrating on tattwas. By awakening tattwas, one develops higher abilities such as clair-voyance, telepathy and intuition. The elements of the earth help to cure diseases and make the body light. Apas tattwa evens out the flow of prana in the body and enables astral travel. Agni tattwa has the ability to turn base metals into precious metals. Vayu tattwa provides knowledge about the past, present and future. Akasha tattwa develops mental projection and reveals metaphysical reality. Despite this, siddhis are not what we strive for in tattwa shuddhi but the purpose is higher spiritual experiences that involve the knowledge of the subtle forces that permeate the entire universe. You thus become more receptive to these forces. You naturally become more intuitive and experience bliss on all levels. In tantric texts one can also read that the knowledge of the elements leads one to freedom from suffering. This is done through the knowledge that all matter is perishable, that the human body is the result of atoms, molecules and energy particles. You stop attaching to things and matter when you know what they consist of - ie. composite energy.

TATTWA SHUDDHI

PERFORMANCE

*Before you start practicing tattwa shuddhi, you and
your teacher/guru should take a sankalpa regarding
how long and how often you should practice. It is said
that a sankalpa should be as short as one day. The person's willpower and mental ability should be taken into
account when determining the time period. A sankalpa
must always be completed. You can start practicing at
any time during the year, but it is said that the period
July-August (shravan) or October (ashwin, the month of
devi worship) gives the best results.*

*You should look after your diet during exercise. Heavy
food makes the body sluggish and slow and is difficult for the body to digest and can make it harder to
be receptive to higher energies. Salt, strong spices and
beverages should be avoided as they increase digestion
and can cause too much acid to form. Light foods are
preferred such as dairy products, fruits and cooked ve-
getables. If you have decided to do tattwa shuddhi daily,
or for some other reason can not keep a light diet, you
should adjust the diet to what is best suited. The special
requirements regarding fasting and diet do not need to
be followed if one does not have a strict sadhana and
only practices tattwa shuddhi once a day.*

According to tradition, tattwa shuddhi should be practiced three times a day. During brahmamuhurta (before sunrise), in the afternoon and during sandhya (dusk). Before the exercise, wash yourself. You should practice in a quiet, calm place with few impressions and sit facing north or east. Before the exercise, light a candle and read out your sankalpa. During the last day, practice mouna and after the last completed exercise, sit and meditate on the formless reality.

Step 1: Preparation.

Practice trataka or pranayama for ten to fifteen minutes before the exercise to calm the mind and go deeper into yourself (pratyahara).

Sit in a comfortable meditation position, close your eyes and practice kaya sthairyam.

Visualize the form of your guru or spiritual guide and feel reverence for him/her.

Take your attention to the Mooladhara chakra and imagine how the Kundalini shakti rises upwards with the sushumna nadi to the Sahasrara chakra on top of the head. Meditate on the mantra So Ham, synchronize with breathing: So on inhalation, from Mooladhara to

Sahasrara and Ham on exhalation from Sahasrara to Mooladhara. Experience the movement of the mantra and the breathing as if it were the movement of your inner consciousness.

Step 2: The creation of tattwa yantras.

Take consciousness to the area between the toes and knees. Visualize the shape of a yellow square which is the yantra for prithvi tattwa, the earth's element. Experience its golden yellow color and weight. At the same time, repeat the bija mantra Lam.

Move your attention to the area between the knees and the navel. Visualize a horizontal crescent moon with two white lotus flowers at each end. The crescent is surrounded by a circle of water. This is the yantra of the monkey tattwa, the element of water. Repeat with the mantra Vam.

Move the attention further to the area between the navel and the heart. Visualize there a red upside-down triangle burning, which is the yantra for agni tattwa, the element of fire. Simultaneously repeat with the mantra Ram.

Now shift your attention to the area between the heart

and the eyebrow center. Visualize a hexagon blue in color, which is yantra for the vayu tattwa. Repeat with the mantra Yam.

Move your attention to the area between the center of the eyebrow and the top of the head. Imagine a circle, the yantra of akasha tattwa, the element of space/ether. In the circle there is shoonya (the emptiness) and it is black or filled with multicolored dots. Repeat the mantra Ham.

Step 3: Resolution of the elements.

Take consciousness back to prithvi yantra. Experience how its form becomes fluid and turns into apas, apas into agni, agni into vayu and vayu into akasha.

Now imagine how the aksha is transformed into its origin, the ahamkara, the ego.

The ego is then transformed into the mahat tattwa, the great principle.

Mahat tattwa dissolves and becomes Prakriti, Prakriti to Purusha (the highest self).

Consider yourself the highest principle, pure and complete.

Step 4: Transformation of the lower nature.

Pay attention to your left side of the abdomen/stomach. Visualize there a small man as big as your thumb. He is called papa purusha. His skin is black as soot, he has glowing eyes and a big belly. In one hand he holds an ax and in the other a shield. He is grotesque in form. You will now transform this man with the help of breathing and mantras.

Hold the right nostril with your right thumb and inhale through the left nostril. At the same time, repeat the mantra Yam four times. Visualize how his face and body transform.

Hold both nostrils. Hold your breath and at the same time repeat the mantra Ram four times. See how the little man is burned to ashes.

Exhale the ashes through your right nostril while repeating the mantra Vam four times. See how the ashes are rolled up into a ball that is mixed with the nectar from the moon in the apas yantra.

Now repeat the mantra Lam. Imagine how the ball on your left side of your stomach transforms into a golden egg.

Repeat the mantra Ham and at the same time visualize how the golden egg grows in size and fills your whole body. It feels like you are born again.

Step 5: Re-formation of the elements.

Reshape the elements in reverse order. From the golden egg you become again the highest principle, Prakriti, mahat tattwa, ahamkara.

From ahamkara you see how akasha yantra is created, from akasha is created vayu, from vayu is created agni, from agni is created apas, from apas is created prithvi.

Locate the area for each tattwa yantra and repeat the mantra for each tattwa as before.

Step 6: Kundalini back to Mooladhara.

When you have recreated all the elements, repeat the mantra So Ham along with the sushumna synchronized with the breathing. Move the attention from Mooladhara to Sahasrara and from Sahasrara to Mooladhara. Experience how you, with the separation of jivatma (your individual soul), separate from paramatma (the cosmic soul). Place jivatma at the heart where its location is.

Visualize the Kundalini shakti that you directed to the
Sahasrara and experience how it returns down to the
Mooladhara through the sushumna while piercing each
chakra on the way down.

Step 7: The shape of the shakti.

Bring your attention to chidakasha. See in front of you
a large, deep sea with a large red lotus flower on the
water. On the lotus flower see the shape of prana Shakti.

Her body is the same color as a sunrise and decorated
with ornaments. She has three eyes and six arms. In her
first hand she holds a trident, in the second a bow made
of sugar cane, in the third a snare, in the fourth a spur,
in the fifth five arrows, and in the sixth a skull with
blood dripping from it.

Keep looking at her beautiful shape and say to yourself
"may she give us happiness".

Step 8: Application of bhasma.

Become aware of yourself sitting on the floor. Become
body conscious. Inhale slowly and deeply. Open your
eyes.

Take some bhasma on the middle and ring fingers and slowly pull the fingers on the forehead from left to right while pronouncing the mantra "Om Hraum Namah Shivaya" or "Om Ham Sa" (Sannyasins).

Take bhasma on your thumb, draw a line from right to left above the other two lines and pronounce the same mantra again.